Toilet Training Tips for Kids with Autism

Shaeri Datta

From the author

Toilet training kids, whether autistic or not, is vital. It will help teach young children the importance of maintaining their hygiene and how to manage themselves. However, traditional methods are often set aside whenever the question of toilet training a child with autism arises.

The amount of information available today on training autistic kids and teaching necessary skills seems to be inadequate.

Much of the information revolves around helping the child learn to remember when to go to the toilet or to notice when they are wet down there.

But did you know: there is no single universal tip or trick to help children diagnosed with autism learn these vital skills.

Rather, multiple factors and different strategies need to be taken into consideration, including but not limited to visuals, routines and prompts.

This highly researched, neatly crafted book aims to provide anyone and everyone who is involved in toilet training autistic kids with a plethora of viable and successful strategies.

This amazing book is a guide to help steer your way to success. Nevertheless, if during the training you hit any training barriers or have any other concerns, feel free to get in touch with me by dropping me an email.

Remember, Toilet Training was and is achievable for every child with autism; albeit success will come in different shapes and sizes.

Shaeri Datta

Email: **shaeri@autismag.org**

Table of Contents

Toilet Training Tips for Kids with Autism 1
A good way to understand the underlying rewards 6
    A way to reward yourself 6
When do you begin toilet training? 8
    Ideal Time 10
    How to Get Started 12
    Visuals 14
    What is a co-active strategy? 15
    Timers 17
A collection of helpful pictographs 19
Visual Sequences 21
Activities 23
Rewards 27
Techniques 30
    Toilet time 33
Accidents 36
    IMPORTANT NOTE ABOUT BATH TIME ACCIDENTS 37
Sensory Issues with Toileting 38
Toileting: Girls' Sensory Issues 41
    Toileting: Boys' Sensory Issues 42
Toilet Timing Sequence 43
    Accident Procedure 43
    Toilet Timing 44
    Bowel Motions 44
Do you find your child insisting on a nappy? A collection of helpful tips: 51
    Sneaky Poo 51

Important and Helpful Tips 53
    Generalizing 54
    Night Time Training 55
The Lurking Dangers of Late Training 57
Social Stories 59
Frequently Asked Questions 61
    My child has learned to hold if his nappy is not on 61
    My child is older than 4 years and shows no signs of toileting 61
    No, my child is unable to comply and cannot imitate. What do I do? 61
    How many bowel movements are ideal for a child every day? ... 62
    My child hates the feel of toilet paper 62
    My child loves unrolling the toilet paper and makes it a mess every time he visits the toilet 62
    My child acts strangely and loves to completely undress during pooing. 62
    My child insists on having nappies to do a poo. 62
    My child's school bus team insists on nappies being on! 62
    When will my child be able to take himself to the toilet? 63
    At times my child has accidents when he is up to his favorite activity. .. 63
    Does a ping pong ball help? 63
    How do I get my child to wipe his own bottom? 63
Tips for Toileting 64
    Keys to Success 66
Conclusion 67
    Success: Its many Shapes and Forms 67

A good way to understand the underlying rewards

It is recommended that before you start toilet training activities, you work out a rough/average estimation of how much nappies will cost you at regular intervals (example: every week).

Once you are ready with the figures, use this saved income to reward yourself, like buying additional accessories that you deem helpful for the benefit of your child.

Many autistic children use an average number of nappies/day. If one calculates a week's expenditure, it could come to as little as 60 to 80 dollars a week. However, if you see the larger picture and calculate for 12 months, the figure comes to a whopping $3,000!

Many of you, including us, will agree that saving $3,000 is not a bad idea.

A way to reward yourself

Use these dollars to do things that will help you stay positive during the course of training. It is a good practice to reward yourself at regular intervals to help you stay right on track.

Some of the ways that you could reward yourself

- Getting a helping hand to do daily chores at home
- Getting yourself spoiled with choices
- Family dinner
- Babysitter or getting a nanny, and much more!

Another way you could spend the $ saved

- Rewarding the child for learning things quickly
- A special toileting seat
- New clothes each time your child completes learning milestones

When do you begin toilet training?

Readiness signs are not always evident in autistic children, unlike their typical peers. One of the subtle signs of being ready is the art of children trying to imitate the actions of others.

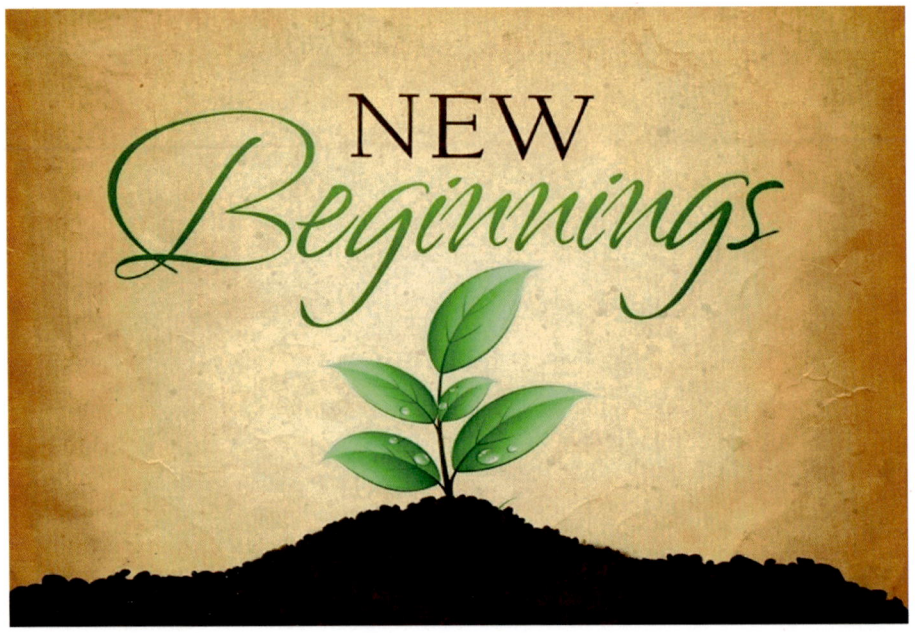

If you see your child doing something that you ask for, this is a sure sign of him/her being ready.

Nevertheless, it is also important to be completely sure that YOU too are ready for the task at hand. Similar to the child, the trainer (in this case YOU, as a parent) needs to dedicate 100% of his/her time.

At times, this can be an emotional drain on the parents. Once you decide it is the right time to begin training, it is good to give yourself some more time to get into the right frame of mind.

Similar to other daily life tasks, toilet training also needs to be done with consistency. For instance, there is no crash course on trying to attain a completely potty trained child in a day or two.

Get everyone at home mentally prepared for the underlying task, even if they won't participate in the course of activities.

For instance, if someone ends up using one nappy on the child during the course of training, the whole process crashes and everything has to begin right from the first step.

Ideal Time

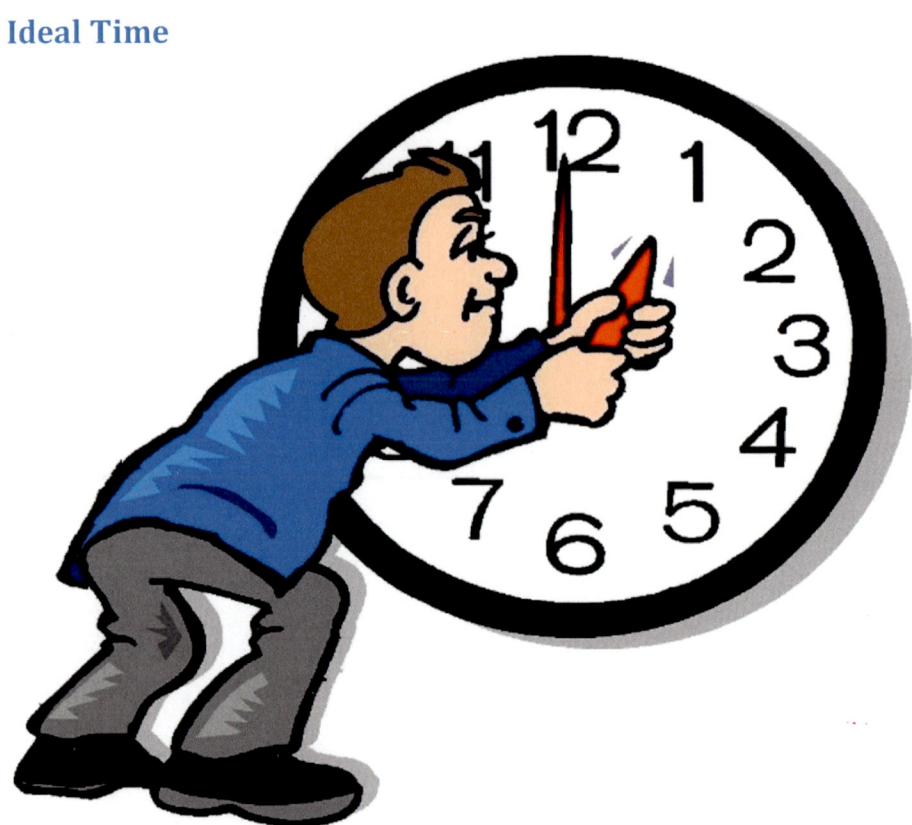

Summer holidays can be a best time to begin your activities. It is usually a good option to start training the first summer after the child turns 3.

A realistic time frame is to allow yourself up to 3 weeks of time before you see improvement.

Although many autistic children are seen to respond within a week's time, some children might take more time.

There have been multiple cases where parents delay their child's potty training until the child is 4 or 5 years, only to be faced by stiff resistance, such as not obliging the commands.

Thus, sticking to a 3-week schedule can help you plan strategies as you progress with the training. During the course of this 3-week activity, it is a good idea to surround yourself with the right people as you may often require additional support.

A mother being interviewed about her toilet training success was asked if they faced any hiccups during the course of training.

She says, "I have older children who were causing disturbances during my stint at training my autistic boy. I failed the first time and requested that my relatives take them on holidays."

She continues, "This helped me hit the right nail and I eventually succeeded the 2nd time."

You too could try strategies such as this if you come across any hiccups during the course of training.

How to Get Started

The best way to start is to keep the end results in mind.

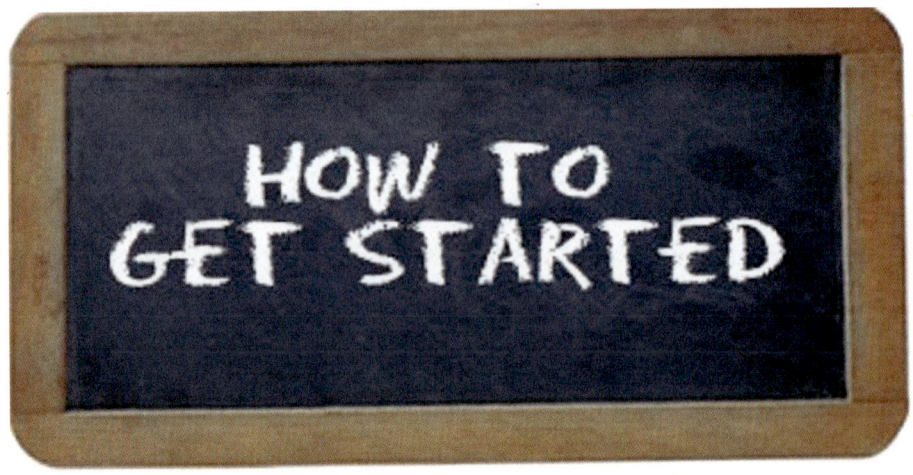

Avoid Potties! Wondering why?

Autistic children at times have issues crop up while generalizing things and the last thing any parent would like is to have the potties being carried around everywhere they go.

Children less than four years old are too young to be able to comfortably sit up on a toilet seat independently. A quick workaround is to have a step stool arranged to help the child independently stand on and make his/her way to the toilet seat.

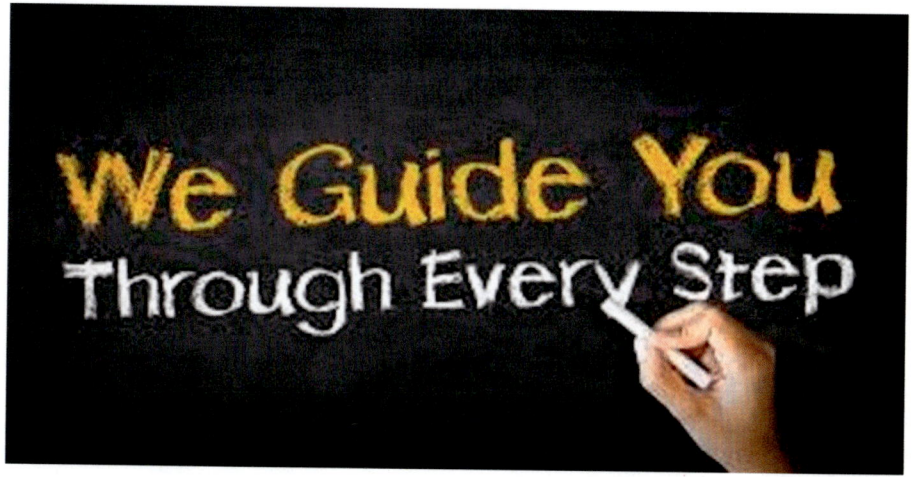

Young children often have weak arms and often struggle to stabilize themselves and avoid falling into the toilet.

To make things easier if you are toilet training a male child, a good option would be to look out for seats with high positioned pieces at the frontal frame that help to ensure that they pee directly into the toilet and do not make a mess on the floor.

Having additional sets of underpants is advisable. Make sure you have a minimum of 10 pairs to be on the safe side. It is advisable to buy additional sets of underpants before you begin potty training.

You can rest assured that each and every penny you spend now will be worth it as you progress through training.

Visuals

Visuals are a great way to help children understand how a process works. It also helps you avoid monotonously repeating things again and again.

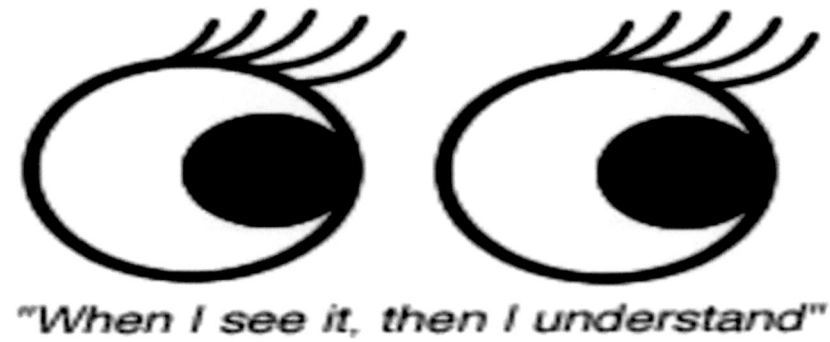

"When I see it, then I understand"

Back here at AutisMag, we know that there is a variety of unique picture symbols that autistic children often find helpful.

Further, we have gone ahead and included a plethora of unique programs to help your child succeed in his/her toilet training mission.

We have tirelessly obtained a large amount from companies involved in designing these useful symbols and we are obliged to give you permission to create the photocopies of these helpful assignments for the purpose of toilet training.

If you have not seen or experienced success with the use of visuals, one trick is to implicate "co-active strategies."

What is a co-active strategy?

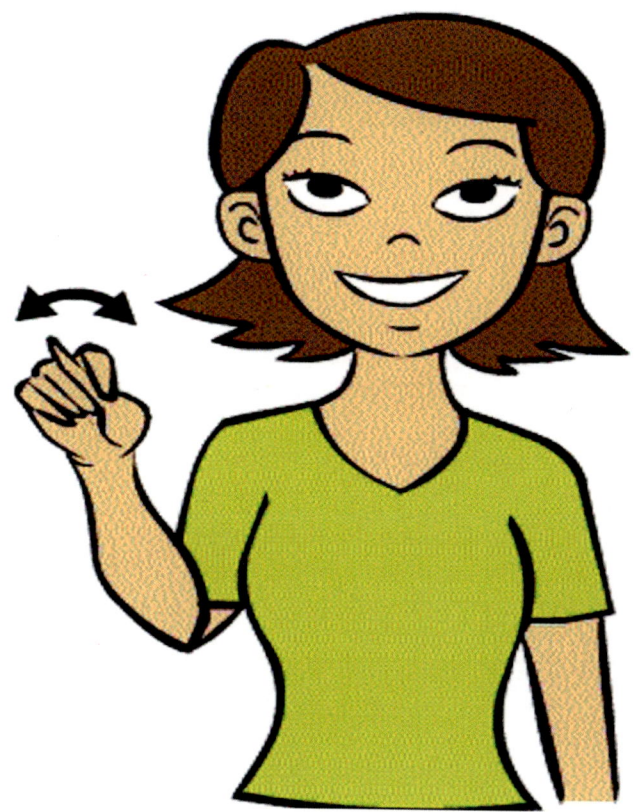

A one-of-a-kind strategy that involves physically guiding your child through the steps while combining your words with action, for instance, you can try saying "pants down," while physically pushing his pants down and holding him.

Another example is when you say "flush the toilet," put your hand on his hand and execute the action together.

Another way is to use sign language. These gestural signs often work miracles and you will be amazed at the gestural consistencies a child will develop.

Nevertheless, it is highly advisable to make sure everyone is on the same page and uses the same form of actions to prevent confusing the child.

Timers

Did you know timers are on the list of must-have tools to achieve greater consistency? These helpful tools can be used not only by adults, but also children who need to be taught their benefits.

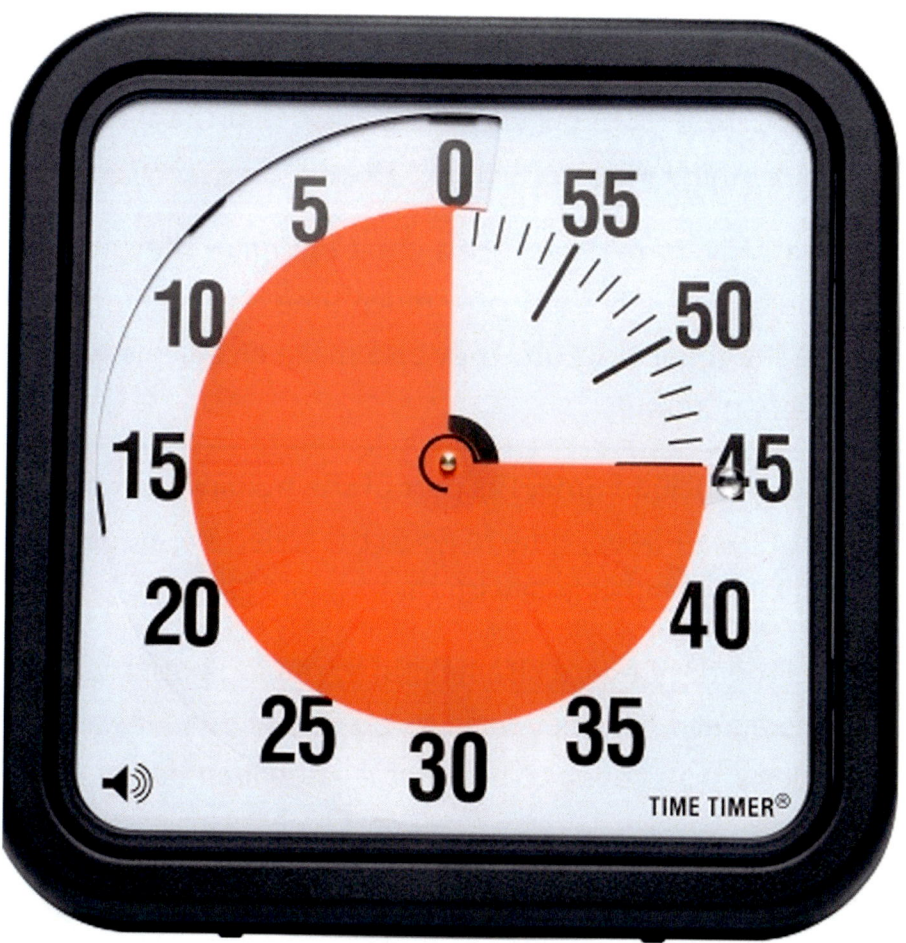

For example, sometimes due to one's busy schedule, it is easy to get distracted or totally forget to take the child to complete his toilet activities.

However, with the timer in place, chances of you missing this important activity are lowered.

There are plenty of timers available on the market. If you do not have one, get one for yourself and you will love it to the core!

However, it is a good practice to shop in a physical store as it helps you understand whether the noise that the timer makes is in sync with your child's taste.

Alternatively, time timers are a great option as they are designed to visually show how much time is remaining before the timer ticks off. They also make an ear-pleasing 'beep-beep' sound.

It is nice to include timers as part of the training routine, for instance: beep-beep, time to go to the toilet. We have seen many children fall in love with their timers being around.

These little devices are also helpful to remind both the child and the adult when they need to get into action. These activities are also seen to be helpful when it comes to eliminating anxiety levels.

A bonus to you as a parent is you can use these devices for your other activities back home to stay organized.

A collection of helpful pictographs

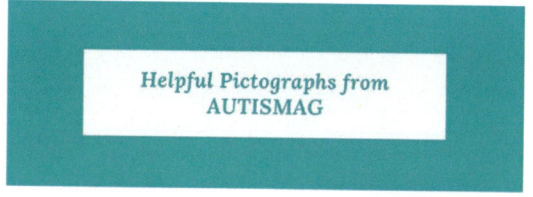

TOILET	UNDERPANTS
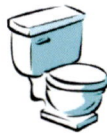	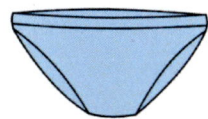
WET	**DRY**
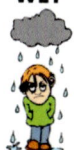	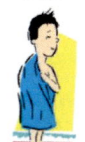
wees	poos
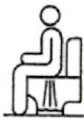	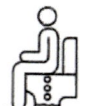
WASH HANDS	**FLUSH TOILET**
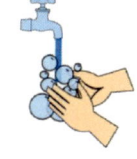	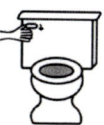
TOILET PAPER	**SIT DOWN**
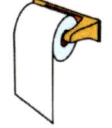	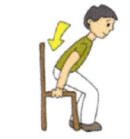
PANTS	**WIPE BOTTOM**
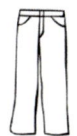	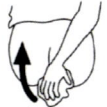

Words	
Toilet	Under Pants
Wet	Dry
Wees	Poos
Toilet Paper	Wash Hands
Flush Toilet	Pants
Sit Down	Wipe Bottom

Visual Sequences

Interestingly, children have been seen to master the art of toileting at a better pace when they are presented with a visual sequence.

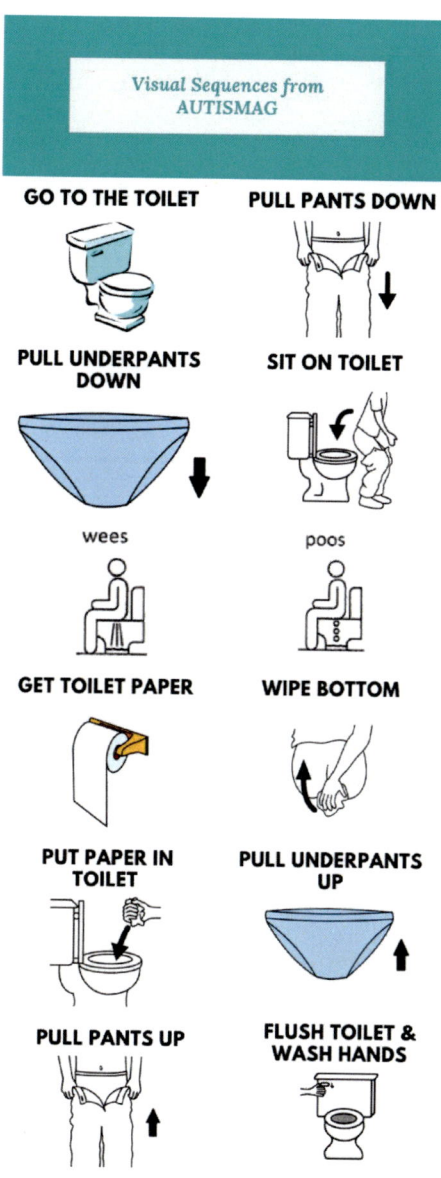

Have the above sequences put on a carefully designed strip and get it laminated.

Next, post this laminated resource next to the toilet seat.

A point worth mentioning: Ensure you have multiple copies of these visuals. It will help you in communicating "toilet time" effectively if you paste these resources at multiple places.

Activities

It is a great idea to prepare a lot of fun activities and execute them you're your children. You will be amazed to learn what all additional things your child will learn with little effort.

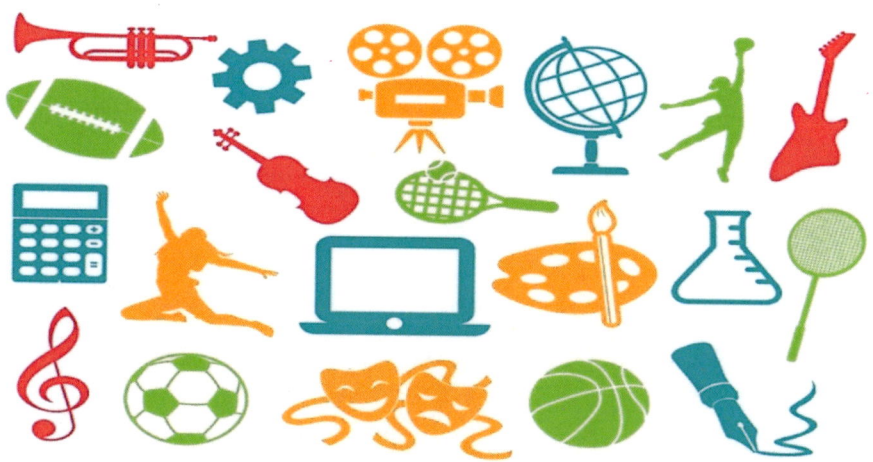

As with the proper notion, treating something with fun takes the pressure off, and the same thing goes with the toilet. When your child starts to enjoy his activities, there is no need to put undue pressure on him or her to carry out the toilet activities.

Wondering how to make his toilet activities a fun task?

Let us help you with simple examples. You may use these or try coming up with your known ideas to help the child perform better.

Get a special kid's train that the child can ride on his way to the toilet. Make sure the child uses this train as a vehicle to reach the toilet. When he finishes his task, make sure he/she doesn't use it for other play activities. This way, the child is forced to use his newfound interest whenever there is bowel pressure.

Another great way is to use a doll or a teddy bear that is placed only next to the toilet seat.

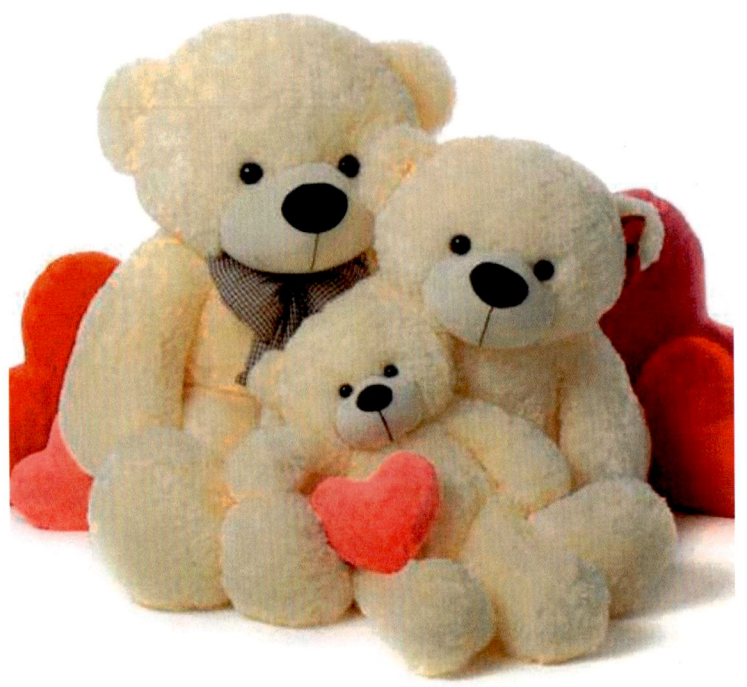

Whenever the kid goes to the toilet, he will be relieved to meet his new friend.

This way you can arouse his interest and make the toilet activity a fun task.

Minnie, a mother, says, "We were advised to carry out a task similar to this by our pediatrician. We bought a DVD player and had it up near the toilet seat. Whenever my kid went to the toilet to relieve himself, he was allowed to watch his favorite show."

She continues, "We found this to be very effective and it solved his poo time problem forever."

David, a father of two autistic children, says, "Initially we had a tough time training our children. We tried many tricks but could not succeed. After some sessions with our trainer, we found our children love the color red. We coated the entire toilet with the color red and since then we have not had an accident back home."

Other notable fun activities include:

Puzzles, books, songs, photos, special interests, and the list goes on!

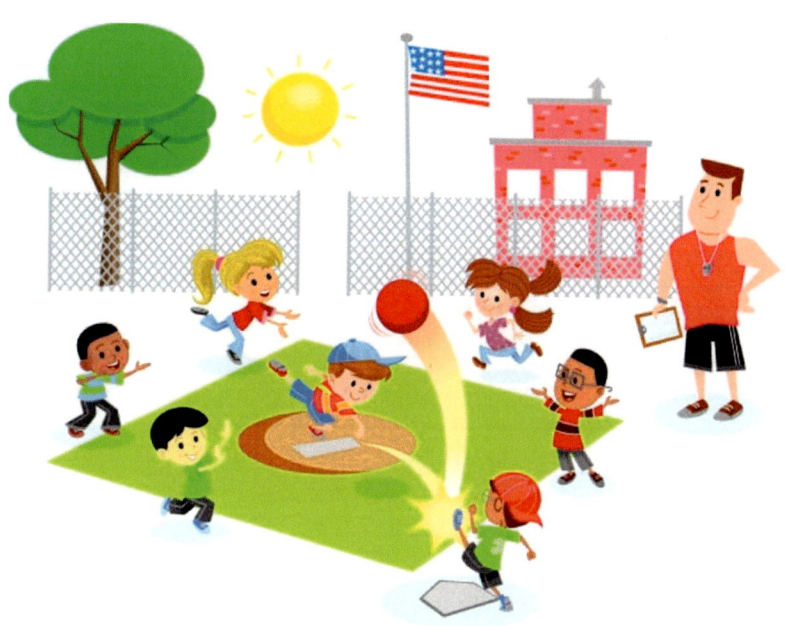

The real key lies in what actually triggers the child.

A few trial-and-error methods are a sure-shot way to redefine your success.

Another helpful but underused resource is GOOGLE. You will find a lot of free interesting activities that many parents have tasted success with. Not only can you use these resources for your success, you can also make a helpful guide or a handy book to help you carry out the activities when you are offline, without putting much thought into remembering what you had browsed through the other day.

Nevertheless, it is always advisable to put the images or other helpful resources that you are utilizing in the toilet areas and make sure the child understands this as an indirect award meant for his timely actions.

If you see your child having trouble with his bowel movements, you can include blowing activities such as blowing fans, air bubbles or blowing candles out, as these are helpful in lightening the pressure.

The blowing activities are helpful in pushing the bowel and it can get into the list of fun activities too. Bathing time also helps with bowel movements.

Rewards

Did you know rewards play an important role not just in training children to achieve something, but also in helping everyone to stay motivated?

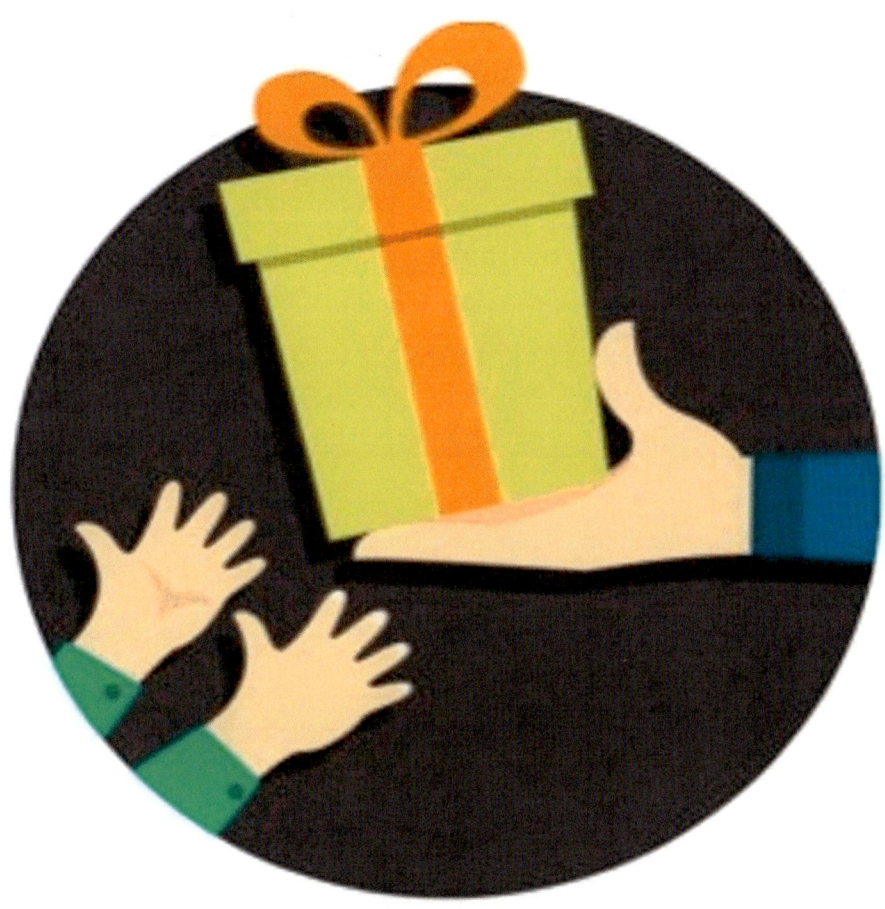

Have you ever pushed yourself hard when you know there are some underlying rewards for your activities?

We believe you have! The same thing works for children too.

Rewards are powerful and they can help you achieve the task in a short amount of time with greater success.

However, the rewards should be instant and powerful.

At times, parents make the mistake of reward withdrawal too soon when they see their child picking up signals. However, it is better to continue rewards till the child picks up his new-found activities as a habit.

Having the reward system fade away slowly and being in sync with the success of training makes sure the level of success remains in tandem as it was.

After you have completely removed the reward system, make sure there is something else that the child finds interesting.

For instance, consider developing a token system and allow the child to pick his/her reward.

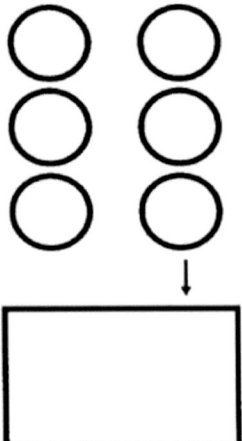

Explain to the child if he sees 5 tokens on the right side of the box, he can have a surprise coming his way.

Further explain if the cards remain on the left side, there are no rewards associated with it. This way, slowly but gradually, you can be sure of minimizing the accidents and getting the child to have a successful nappy-free time.

Make sure you set the number of tokens to be put on the right side in an appropriate manner that varies case to case.

For instance, there are children who require the toilet as many as 10 times a day. On the other hand, there are children who use the toilet seat for just a few times a day, maybe 3 to 4 times. It is important to work out what is right for your child.

A helpful tip: Always remember that rewards can wear out. Change your rewarding tricks in a timely manner and retain the positives of the learning.

Techniques

During the start of any training, a fair degree of intensity needs to be in place to measure success during the first few days. A measurable time frame is 1 to 3 days.

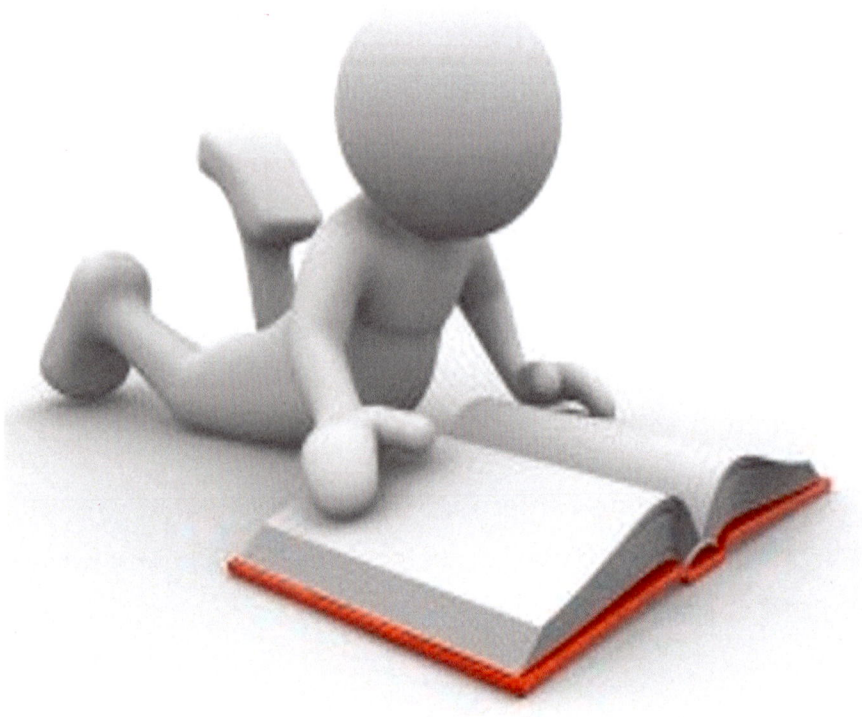

In the worst case scenario, a child needs to understand the sensation of going to the toilet within a week's time of starting the training.

Nevertheless, the intensity of the training has to be taken into account with other notable factors that define the course of success.

For instance:

- Compliance
- Age
- Low or high functioning
- Sensory issues

At times, higher functioning autistic children will not need an increased level of intensive training. Station yourself right inside or next to the toilet! More often than not, bathrooms with an attached toilet are seen to be the best places for training a child.

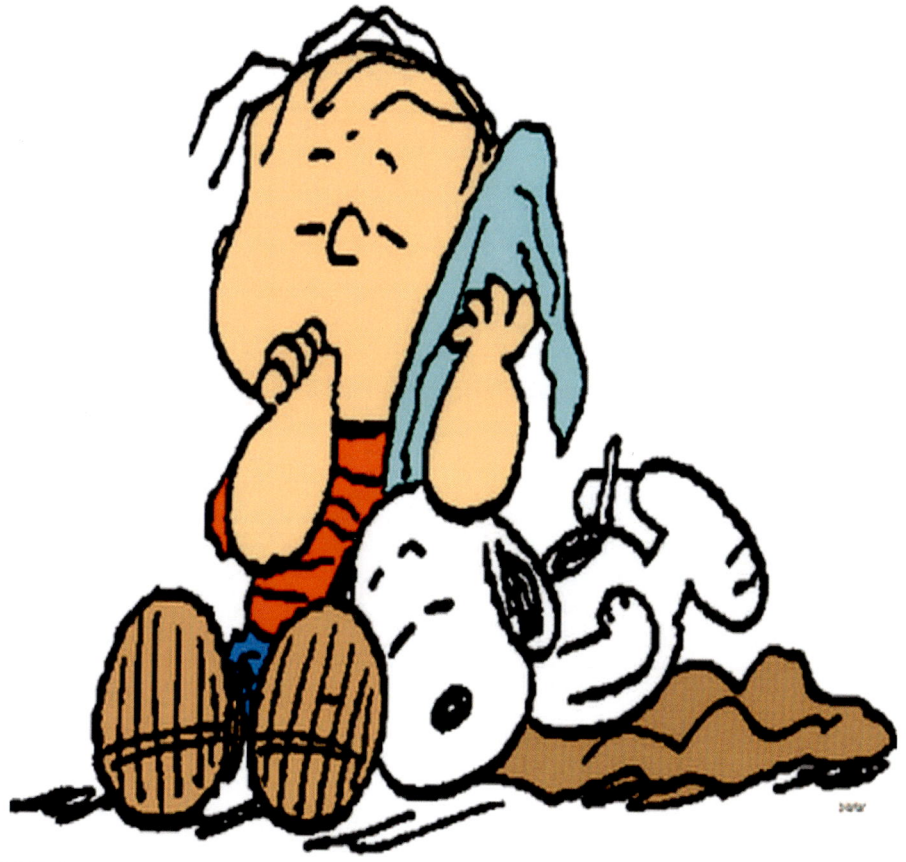

Make sure the child is comfortable during the course of his training. Have the nappies removed once you begin your training sessions!

Make sure the child doesn't use a nappy during the course of the day and put nappies on when the child goes to bed to avoid bedwetting.

If you leave the child with the nappy on during the day, the child will learn to control his bowel movements until he is in it, which ideally should not be the case.

For instance:

- Compliance
- Age
- Low or high functioning
- Sensory issues

At times, higher functioning autistic children will not need an increased level of intensive training. Station yourself right inside or next to the toilet! More often than not, bathrooms with an attached toilet are seen to be the best places for training a child.

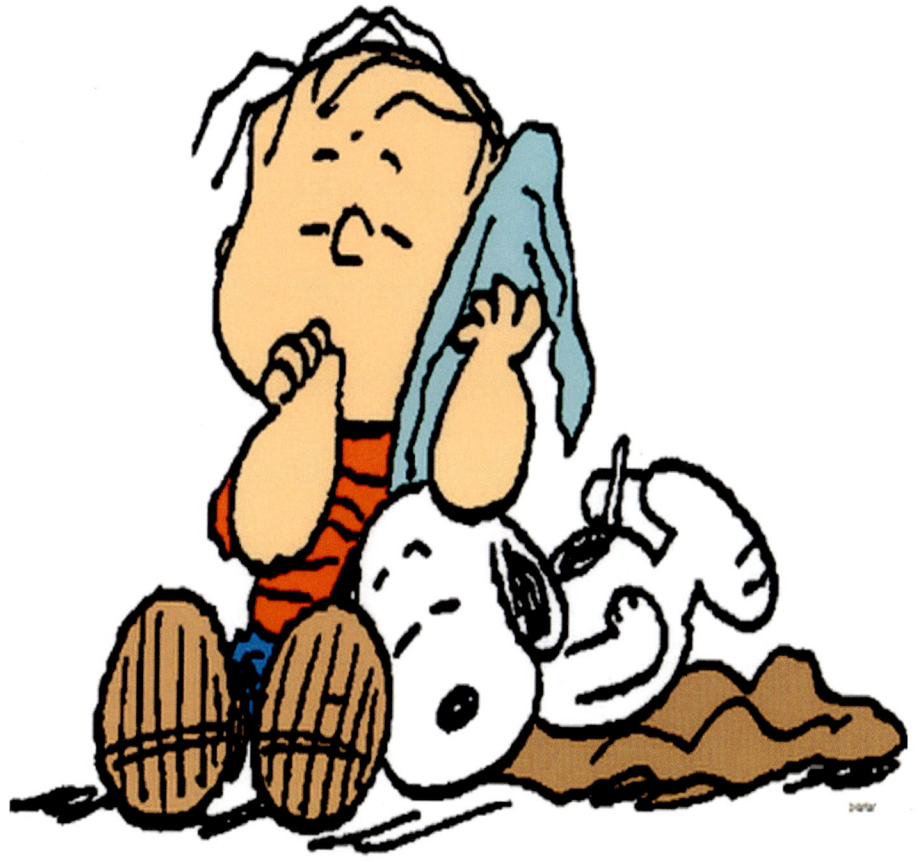

Make sure the child is comfortable during the course of his training. Have the nappies removed once you begin your training sessions!

Make sure the child doesn't use a nappy during the course of the day and put nappies on when the child goes to bed to avoid bedwetting.

If you leave the child with the nappy on during the day, the child will learn to control his bowel movements until he is in it, which ideally should not be the case.

Toilet time

Put the child on the hot seat once every half an hour (30 minutes). Make sure toilet seat time is no longer than 10 minutes. As the child increases his awareness about the toilet seat, slowly start increasing the interval time from 30 minutes to one hour.

This way, you can slowly but surely increase the success of the toileting routine. Alternatively, give the child enough fluid to trigger his/her toilet-going time. *Remember, smaller steps lead to faster success.*

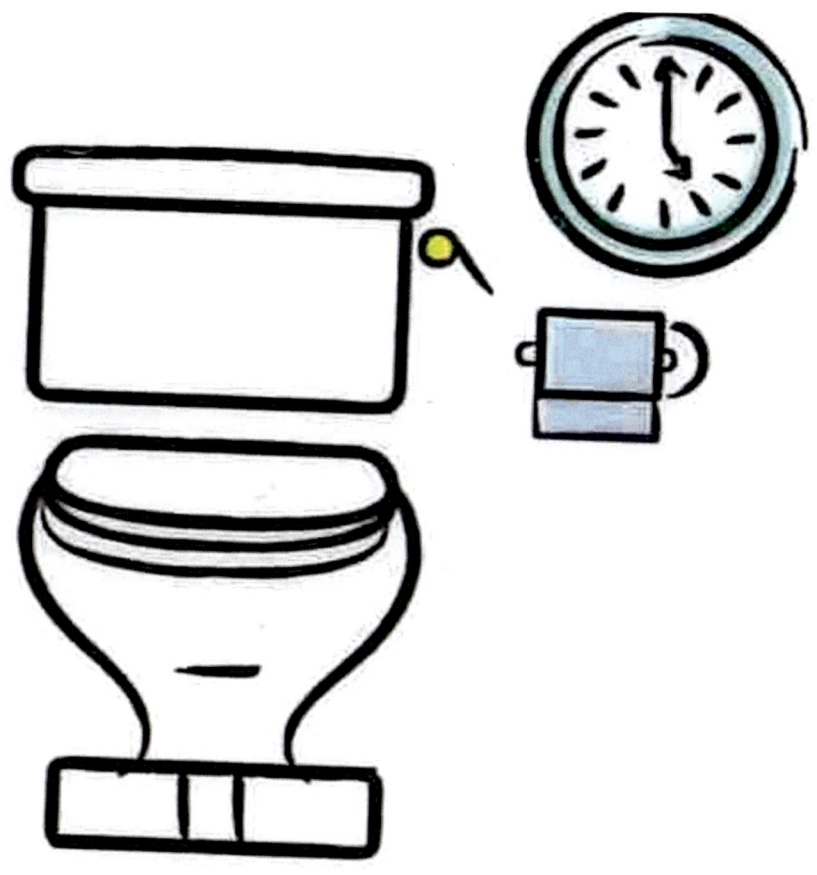

As you eventually progress, success will come in its own shape and form.

And do not stop rewarding the child, even if you have to do it multiple times. Keeping rewards small helps you to not burden your pocket.

As you go on, all of a sudden the child makes the right choice between his poo and pee.

After the child has tasted smaller successes, slowly move them away from the toilet and the bathroom and help them slowly integrate into the natural environment.

You will be surprised at the way your child comes back to you whenever he faces pressure inside to relieve himself.

If possible, consider recording all the instances during the course of training. It will help you create memories that you can cherish many years down the line.

Teach the child each and every step that is a part of toilet training, for instance, the necessity of putting on underpants, washing hands, and flushing the basin after use.

During the course of each step, observe whether the child is grasping as he should or if he has any trouble in doing so. If you find he has trouble in grasping things, an ideal strategy is to break down the task further and slowly work your way up.

It is always a good habit to start things with an end goal in mind. Once the child learns all the steps, you can consider rewarding yourself something of your taste. After all, much of the credit goes to you for tirelessly putting things in the right order.

Accidents

Many parents wonder if their children are trying to be naughty when they have accidents. It should be noted that an accident is neither bad nor naughty.

An accident is an accident.

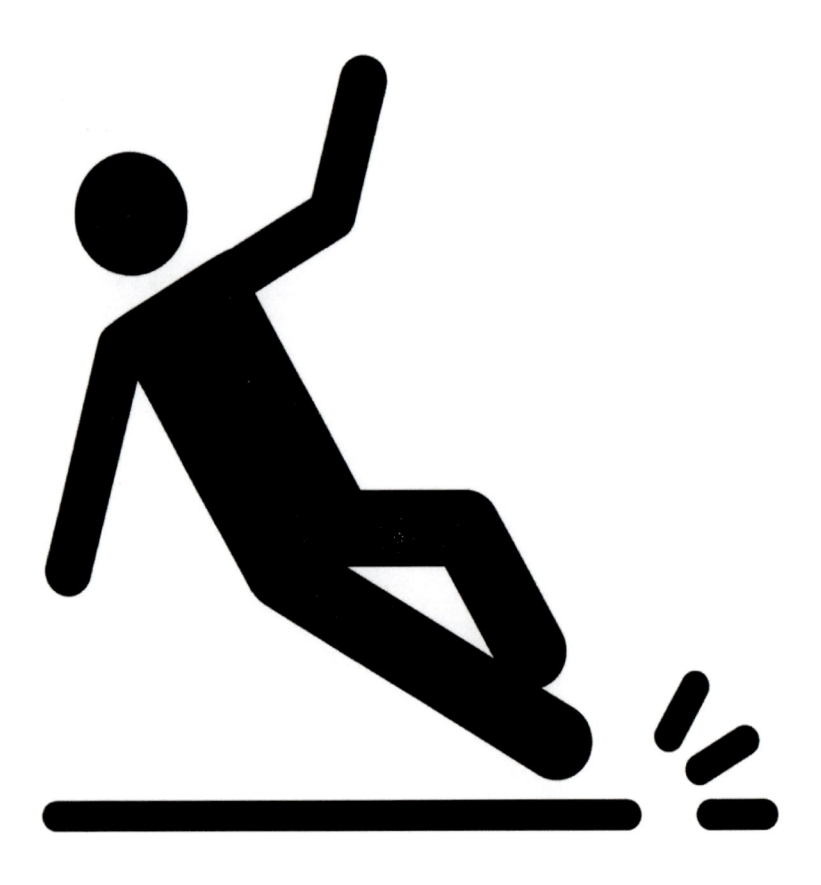

Be careful how you react when your child has an accident. Many times, parents make the mistake of being over-reactive which results in a child losing all of his learned skills.

Autistic children are often seen to have an innate fear of failure and this could hamper their ability in a much bigger way.

Avoid using the word "NO" too often. Instead, you can consider modeling what they should actually have done.

For instance, instead of saying, "Oh you have wet pants" and shouting, "YOU NEED TO USE THE TOILET," consider saying "let us clean what you have already done and try out the same thing with dry pants."

Your approach to how you react makes a big difference while training. Another helpful tip is to get the child to do the clean-up along with you. Afterwards, have them wash their hands thoroughly, signifying the importance of washing hands after toilet time.

IMPORTANT NOTE ABOUT BATH TIME ACCIDENTS
If you find your child weeing or pooing in the tub, it is important for you to explain that wees and poos are done in the toilet and not while having a bath. Be consistent with your explanation.

Sensory Issues with Toileting

At times, some children are seen to have sensory issues crop up during the course of their toilet training. It is highly critical to respect their sensory sensitivities and it is something that should not be ignored, but rather worked upon.

Sensory issues are seen to include a wide range of areas. Hypo- and hyper-sensitivity are both a part of a child's sensory movement. Touch sensory issues is seen to be a challenging issue most of the time.

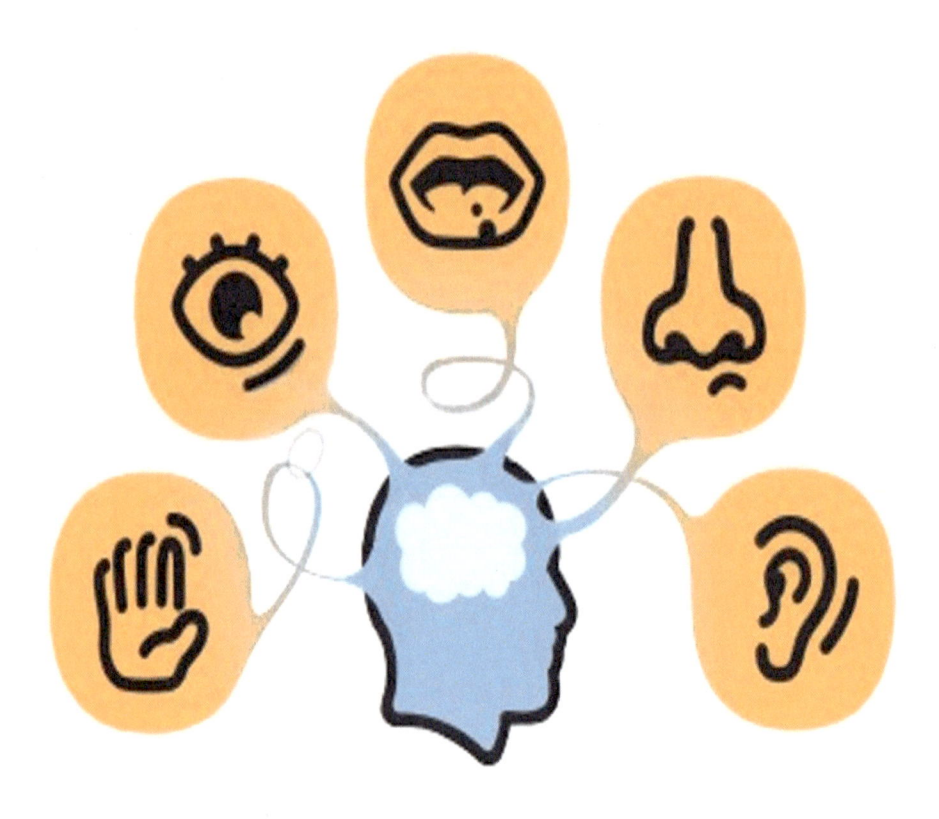

Many autistic children are seen to have touch issues that revolve around toileting.

At times, there are some children who do not notice being wet, while on the other hand, there are children who have deeper touch issues ingrained in them.

Below highlighted are some of the sensory considerations:

- Smell (toilet sprays, bowel motion)
- Taste
- Touch
- Sound
- Looks
- Movements
- Visual Lights

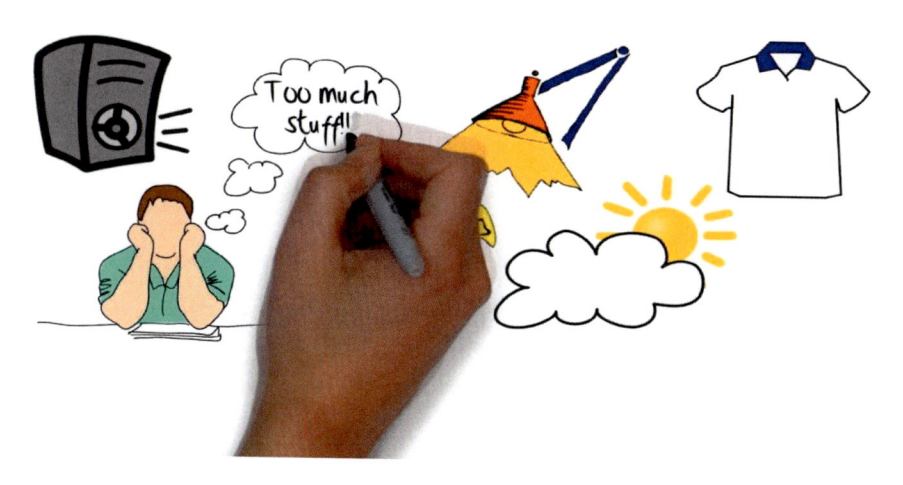

If you find your child loving the heavy feel of a wet nappy, you can consider switching his nappies to thicker nappies available on the market.

Examples of Sensory Issues with Toileting

If you are not sure about selecting the right toilet seat for your child, occupational therapists can help you sort out the issue.

There are many toilet seats that are designed to help those with specific needs. For instance:

- Toilet seat cover
- Special step
- Toilet insert
- Seatbelt

These seats are designed with one aim: To help children be secure.

Toileting: Girls' Sensory Issues

Underwear is seen to annoy some autistic girls.

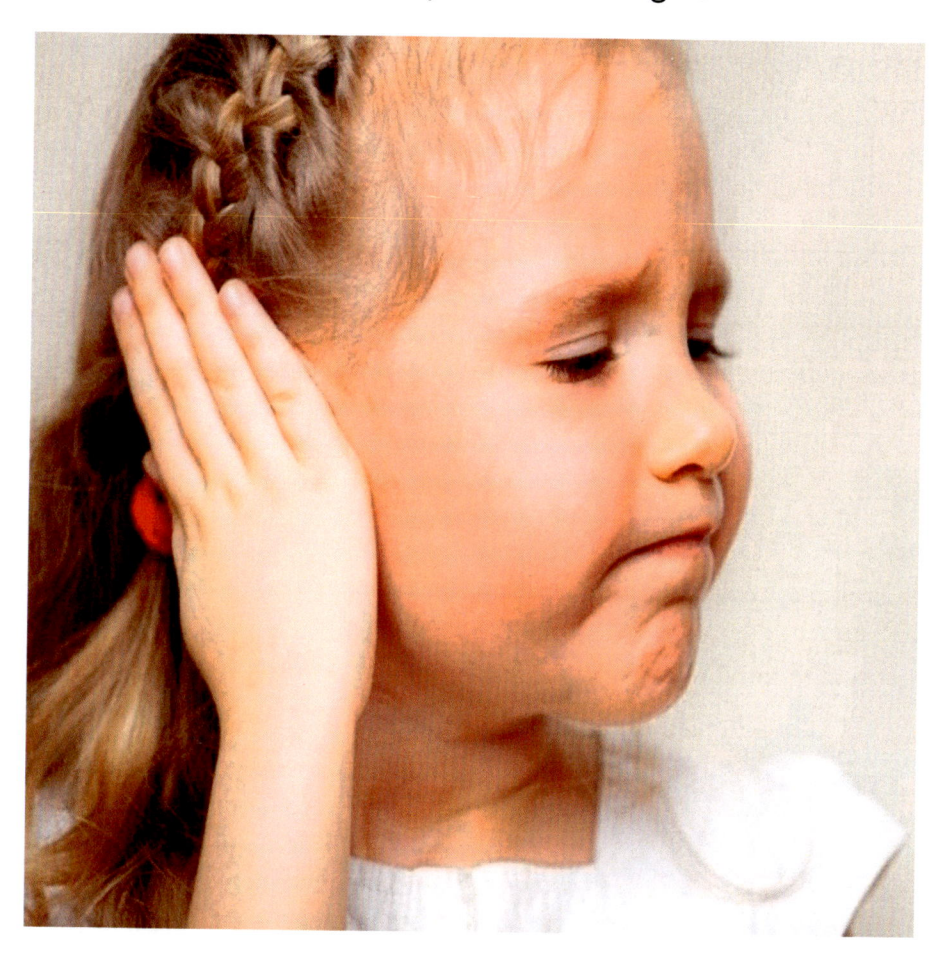

A good alternative can be using bike shorts with nothing worn underneath

(This can work wonders for girls who do like the feel of deep pressure.)

Toileting: Boys' Sensory Issues

Learning to wee standing up is an easy task for the majority of the male population.

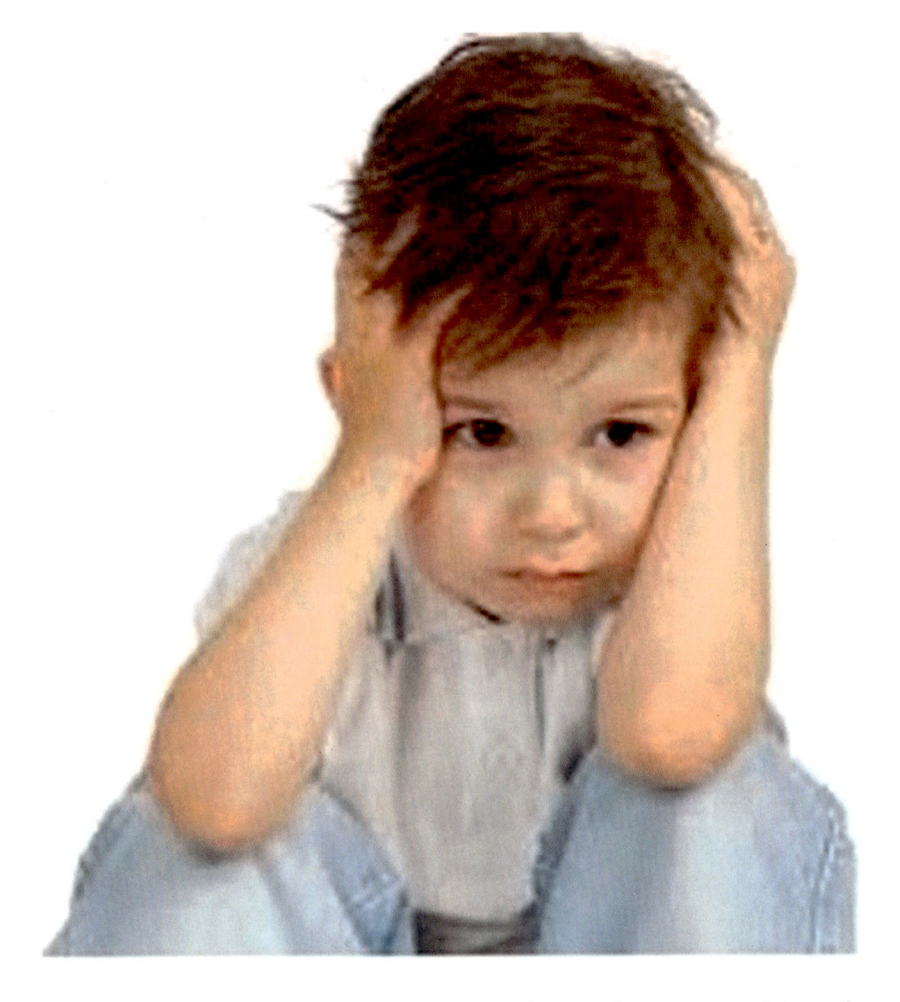

However, sitting and performing the task is something that should be learned.

You can train your child to look up to the seat, having their feet off the ground, and help them perform their tasks in the right way.

Toilet Timing Sequence

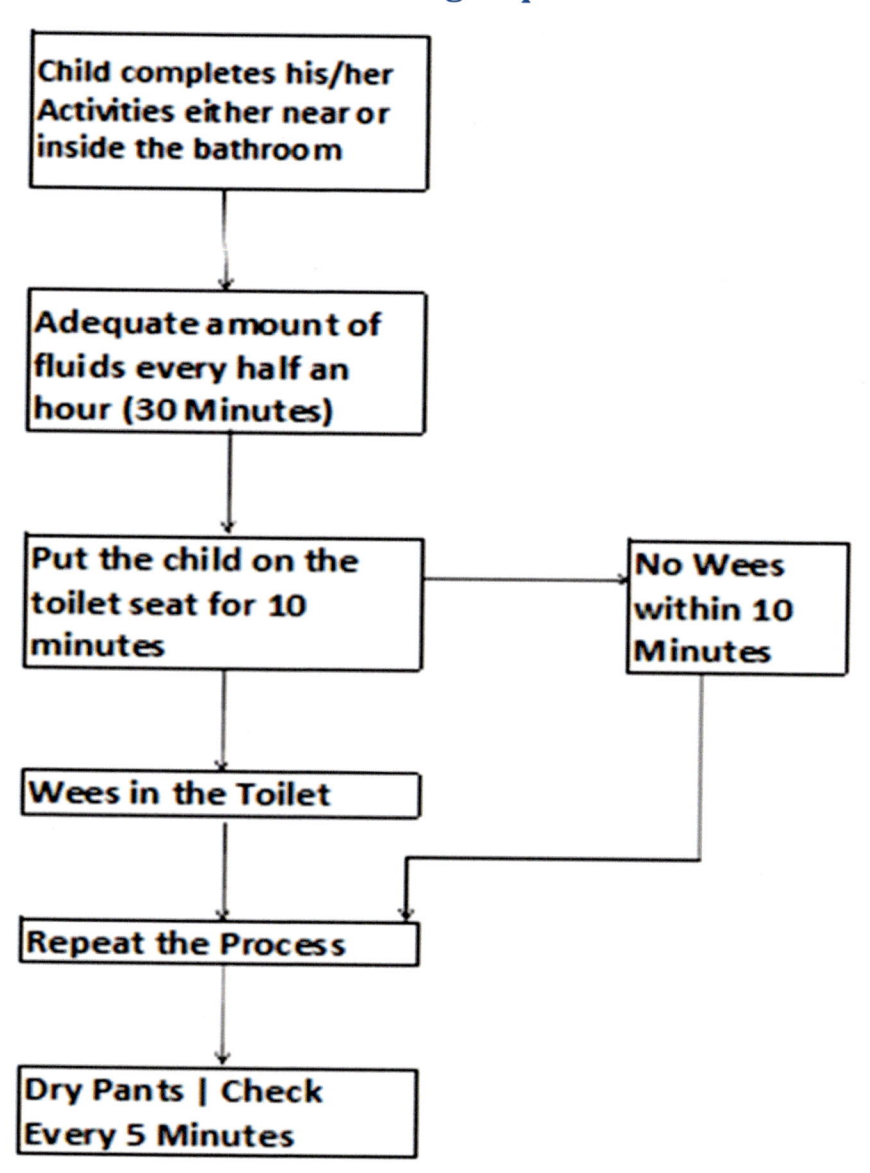

```
┌─────────────────────────┐
│ Child completes his/her │
│ Activities either near or│
│ inside the bathroom     │
└────────────┬────────────┘
             ↓
┌─────────────────────────┐
│ Adequate amount of      │
│ fluids every half an    │
│ hour (30 Minutes)       │
└────────────┬────────────┘
             ↓
┌─────────────────────────┐       ┌─────────────┐
│ Put the child on the    │──────→│ No Wees     │
│ toilet seat for 10      │       │ within 10   │
│ minutes                 │       │ Minutes     │
└────────────┬────────────┘       └─────────────┘
             ↓
┌─────────────────────────┐
│ Wees in the Toilet      │
└────────────┬────────────┘
             ↓
┌─────────────────────────┐
│ Repeat the Process      │
└────────────┬────────────┘
             ↓
┌─────────────────────────┐
│ Dry Pants | Check       │
│ Every 5 Minutes         │
└─────────────────────────┘
```

Accident Procedure

- During an accident, get the attention of the child by saying aloud, "Oh, look! You wet your pants!"

- Have your child feel his wet pants
- Make sure the child is involved in the clean-up activity when accidents happen.
- Have the child take off his/her pants after accidents and make him put them into the bucket.
- Instruct the child to clean the pants and put them on.
- Have the child perform his toilet activities again, but this time in the toilet.
- Return to your regular training activities.
- Start giving your child ample amounts of fluids again.

Toilet Timing

Create good and achievable routines while working on toilet time. Fix/set the times when you expect your child to use the toilet. For instance:

- When they are up in the morning
- Each time they leave home
- Before bed
- If you believe your child won't have access to a toilet seat for a couple of hours due to some activity
- Before eating
- Before getting into water (for bathing, swimming, etc.)

Bowel Motions

The hardest thing to achieve during the course of training is to train a child to poo in the correct order. If you are facing a hard time getting your child accustomed to poo training, it would be worth noting that you are not alone.

Many parents have undergone difficulties in striking the right chord. Further, it would be worth mentioning many children find the poo training experience disgusting and it makes them learn something out of their comfort zones.

Thus it is highly advisable to have your nerves in place and maintain enough calmness while you work your way to success.

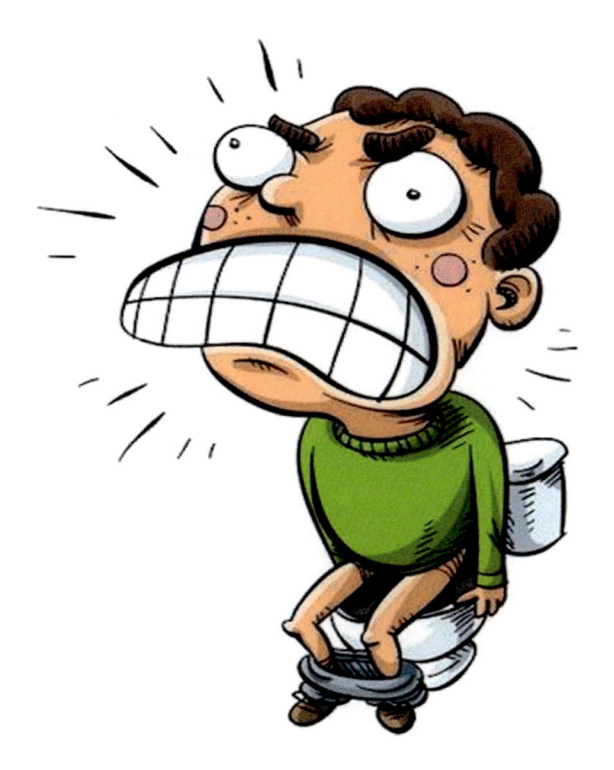

Many autistic children are known to have bowel complexities and anybody training a child should take this into consideration.

The best advice we at AutisMag have is to patiently decode your child's bowel pattern. For instance, a mother recollects that her child used to have his poo time just before retiring to bed.

Her child used to have a strange gaze just before it was about to happen. Initially, she was unsure if she had detected the right pattern.

Nevertheless, she tried this trick as per AutisMag's suggestion. Today, she is elated to have her child completely trained.

Eliza, a trainer, says, "During the course of training my young clients, I have found a trick that works like a breeze. I wait until the child is just about to poo and I quickly put them onto the toilet seat. I have observed children gradually beginning to get accustomed to using the potty during their poo time."

When Eliza was questioned on how she manages to note the exact time when the child was about to poo, she explains, "I maintain a strict observation checklist and leave children to soil their pants for a week.

Once I get hold of the pattern, I dive right in there and achieve the results without much fuss."

Children get accustomed to nappies right from their birth. They easily learn to manage to poo in their nappy or to hold on without pooing if they are without one.

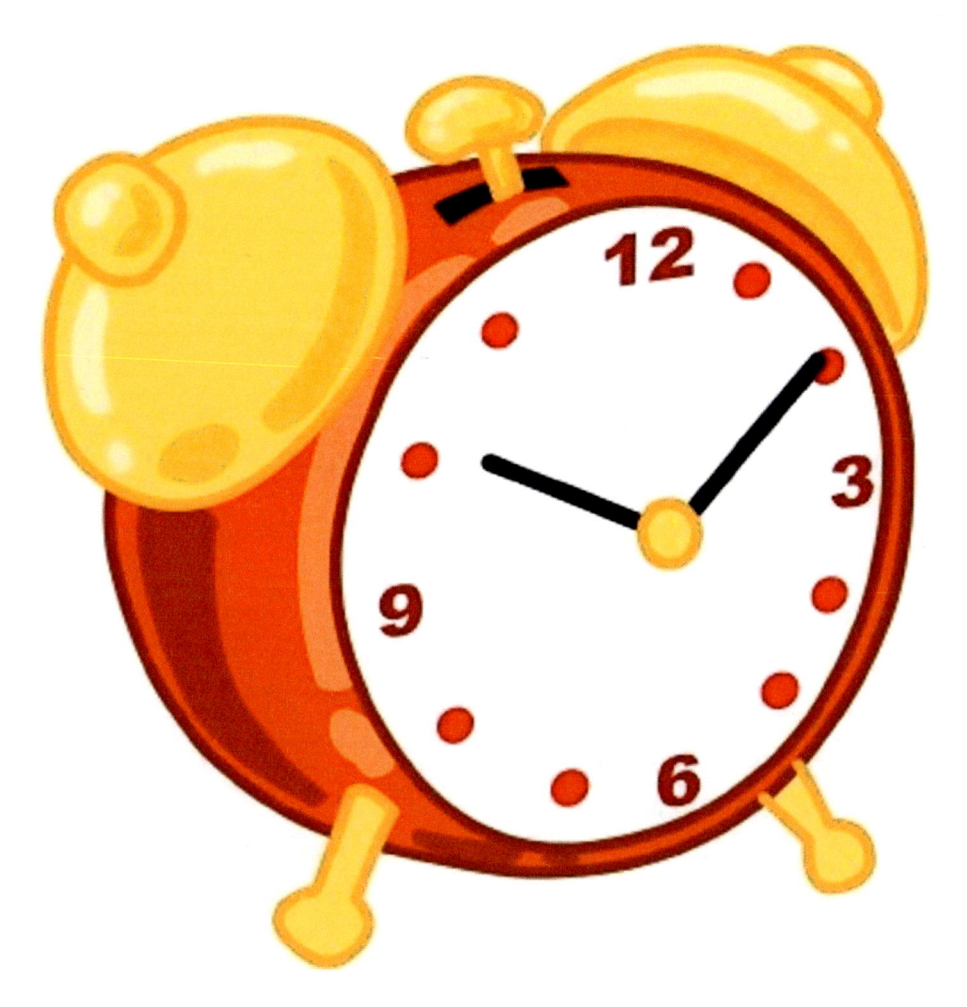

Eliza says, "I had a difficult time with one child who refused to poo in the toilet despite trying each and every trick up my sleeve. The child went straight for eight days, refusing to poo. However, on the ninth day, she could no longer control and passed her bowels in the toilet."

She further continues, "After this episode, the child has no longer had an accident, as she now knows what is expected out of her."

"At times, it pays large dividends if one is ruthless in their training," explains Eliza.

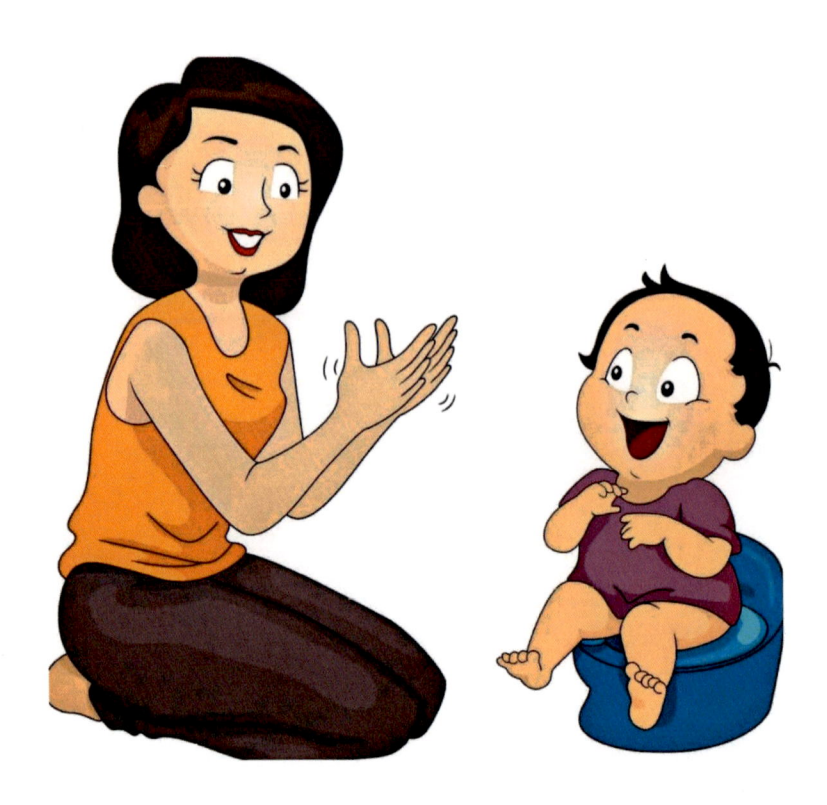

It is always great to reward a child for any poo attempt. Once they have achieved their success, reward them heavily.

It should be well noted that poo accidents should never be treated in the same way as wee accidents. Autistic children are often seen to be poo smearers.

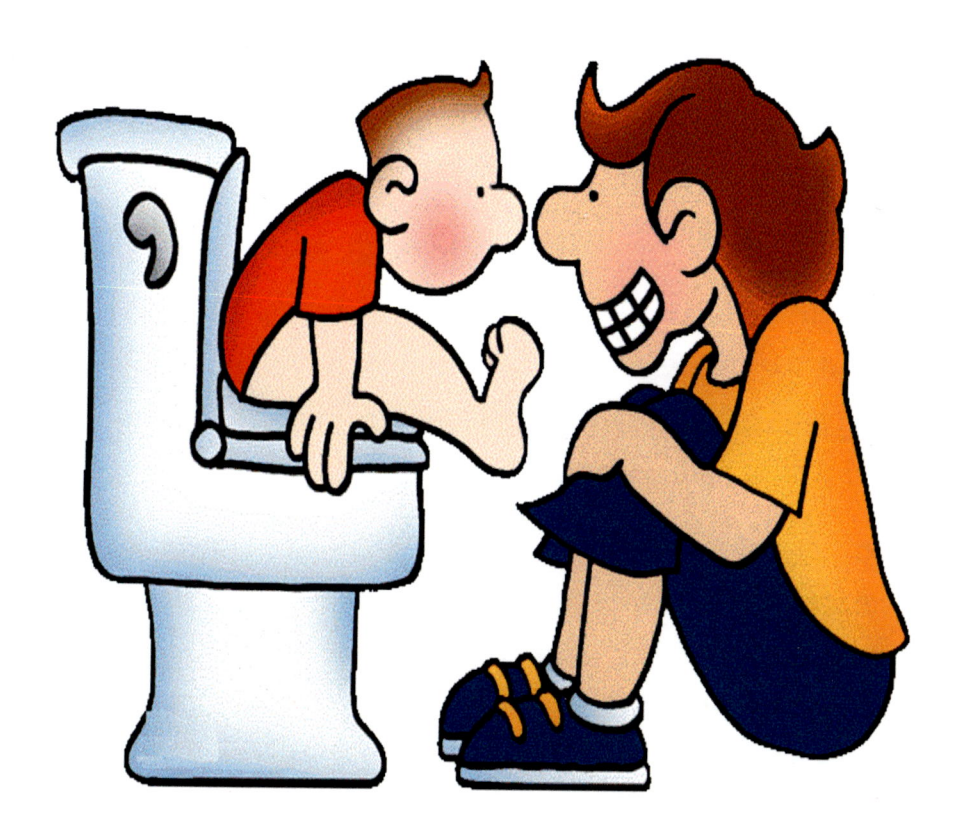

Touching poos should be discouraged, no matter what!

Always put the child on the seat and tell them poos are something that goes inside the toilet and is not meant to be played with.

Use an aggressive social story build up and make them watch videos that highlight what necessary steps have to be taken in order to avoid these unfavorable situations.

Below are some unique strategies that are known to help children as well as their parents in getting the task done.

Alternatively, there is an age-old saying when it comes to using unique strategies, "Execute the strategy no matter how bizarre it may seem."

Have a look at some of the tricks that have worked wonders for many parents:

Have the toilet area painted in a color that your child loves. An autistic boy was too scared to use the toilet. Once the toilet was painted red, the child enjoyed his toilet time. The child was in love with the red color.

Another child, a little girl, showed bouts of depressive symptoms when her nappy was removed. Her trainers worked out a unique way of making her sit on the toilet while having a wide hole in her nappy. This trick worked wonders.

Get as many pairs of underwear as possible; the child might need many in the initial phase of training.

It is well worth mentioning that sitting for longer periods of time when pooing than weeing is quite different and normal.

At times, depending on the situation you may need to increase the time a child has on the toilet. One should always remember distractions help increase time on the toilet.

Do you find your child insisting on a nappy? A collection of helpful tips:

Observation plays a great role.

Have you ever observed how your child poos? Do you find him/her to be sneaking under the table?

- If so, your child might need some dark and private place to poo in peace. You can work around this by switching the toilet lights off and leaving them on their own for a while.
- If you find your child trying to squat while pooing, try to have his/her feet elevated while being seated on the toilet.
- If you find your child leaning on the bed while pooing, it signals they might need something to hold onto while pooing.
- If you find your child getting immersed in some of their favorite activities, it might signify calmness. Try to get this situation inside the toilet and you will be amazed at how quickly and easily you can achieve results.

Sneaky Poo

If you find your child's pants with little bits of poos, it might signify a constipation problem. Wait for things to get normal before starting toilet training activity.

If you repeatedly see bits of poos in his pants, it might signal constipation complexities.

Seek medical assistance if you see your child has a constipation problem.

The doctor has a bigger role to play in ensuring the big, hard poo is moved out. Once done, and with timely medication, the child can be brought back to normal. Once done, the child should be made to learn his/her poos no longer hurt.

Important and Helpful Tips

Cloth soiling is not done on purpose and the child usually doesn't know his mistake. It should be well understood that the children should never be blamed for soiling their pants and it is not their fault.

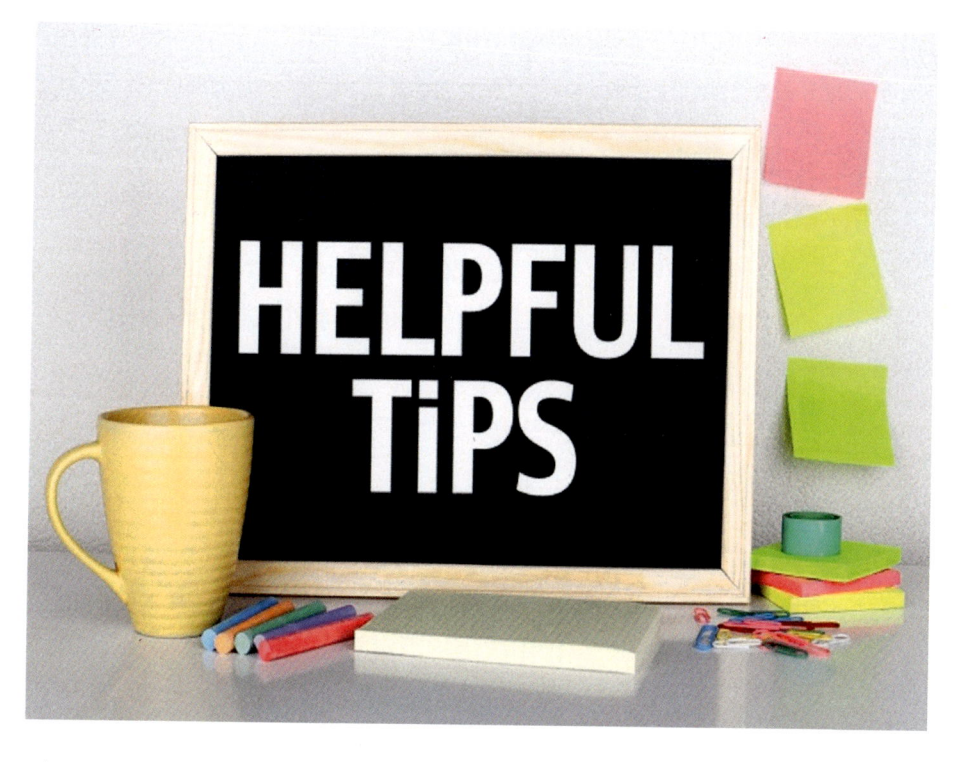

Always remember, things started going out of control because the child was getting hurt while he had constipation problems.

Note that your child is not trying to be manipulative or trying to hurt you.

Never get angry at children for things that they have no control over. It will only complicate things and they will have hard time learning.

Make poo time a relaxing and fun activity and encourage the child to sit as long as he wants to relieve himself completely.

Try searching for additional helpful tips on the internet and you will be amazed to see how people have overcome their children's sneaky poo problems.

Generalizing

Autistic children have trouble generalizing and toilet training is no different. Often, generalizing in the right way and direction is one of the hardest things to achieve during the course of toilet training.

Always make sure you have the toileting sorted out first before resorting to any form of generalizing. However, remember generalization too is a part of training activities.

At times, you will see your child has generalization problems while going to a different toilet, even within the home, and is happy to stick with the toilet where he began his training.

Be patient and continue his training, but this time making him go to different toilets once he has succeeded in his initial toilet training task. Remember, your child has been using nappies for a long time and is accustomed to using them. It may take a while for the child to take control of his new habits.

Night Time Training

Everyone reacts differently to night time training. Some children go dry during the nights as with the days without any fuss. On the other hand, some children will take years together to master the night time training activity. Remember, there is nothing normal or abnormal about this situation.

Neurotypical children too at times take years to master the art of not wetting their beds during night time.

A natural instinct of a human body is to go off or shut down as the night befalls. However, some people need to learn this and might take extra time to master this.

Often, night time training takes place according to its own pace and bed wetting shouldn't be stressed about until the child reaches the age of six.

If you find your child refusing to put on a night time nappy, the following tips offer you some helpful advice:

- It pays to invest in good plastic-backed sheet mattresses or blankets. Invest your saved money on getting quality sheets so that you need not dry the bed every day.
- Stop giving any fluids when the clock hits 6 or 7 PM. You can tune in the correct time before the child goes to bed. Stop fluid intake around 5 hours before bedtime.

- Use social stories about the importance of being dry in bed while you put your child to sleep.
- Make sure the child uses the toilet before going to bed even if they resist.
- Another helpful tip is to put a nappy on one hour after they go to bed. After that, wake them up and take them to the toilet. Put the nappy on. Gradually increase the hours until they are completely nappy-free.
- As soon as the child wakes up, make it a habit to have the night nappy removed and take them to the toilet.
- Repeat the above steps until they become a normal part of the daily routine.

The Lurking Dangers of Late Training

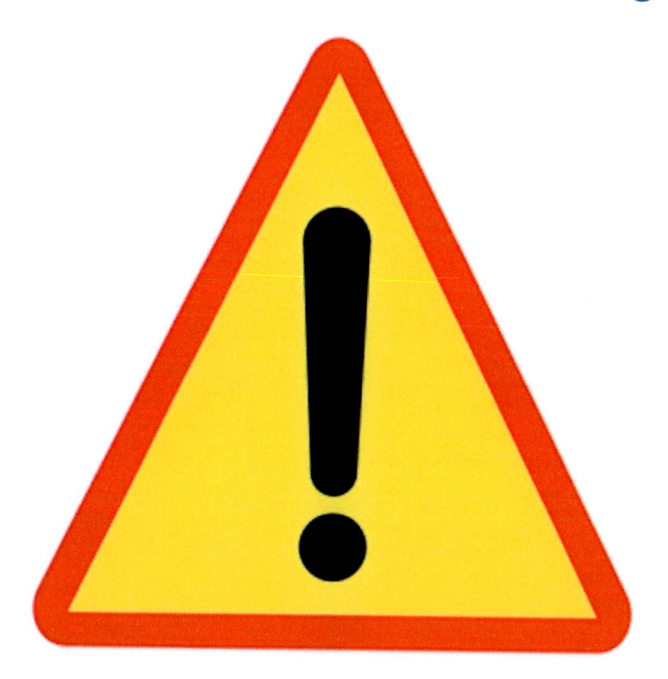

It is important to train children on basic hygiene activities as soon as possible. If children are left too long in nappies they might end up not achieving the required muscle growth for toileting.

If you choose to have the training delayed, it is better to start by at most age 4.

If your child is older, start the training without a second thought and do not wait for summer to arrive.

You should always remember, the aim of toilet training is not to watch out for any readiness signs. Rather the aim should be to strike the right toilet timing.

If your child is over five years old, you need to have higher levels of persistence to make them learn things. You might further require more regular toilet times to teach older children.

Social Stories

Carol Gray is touted to be the main person behind the concept of social stories.

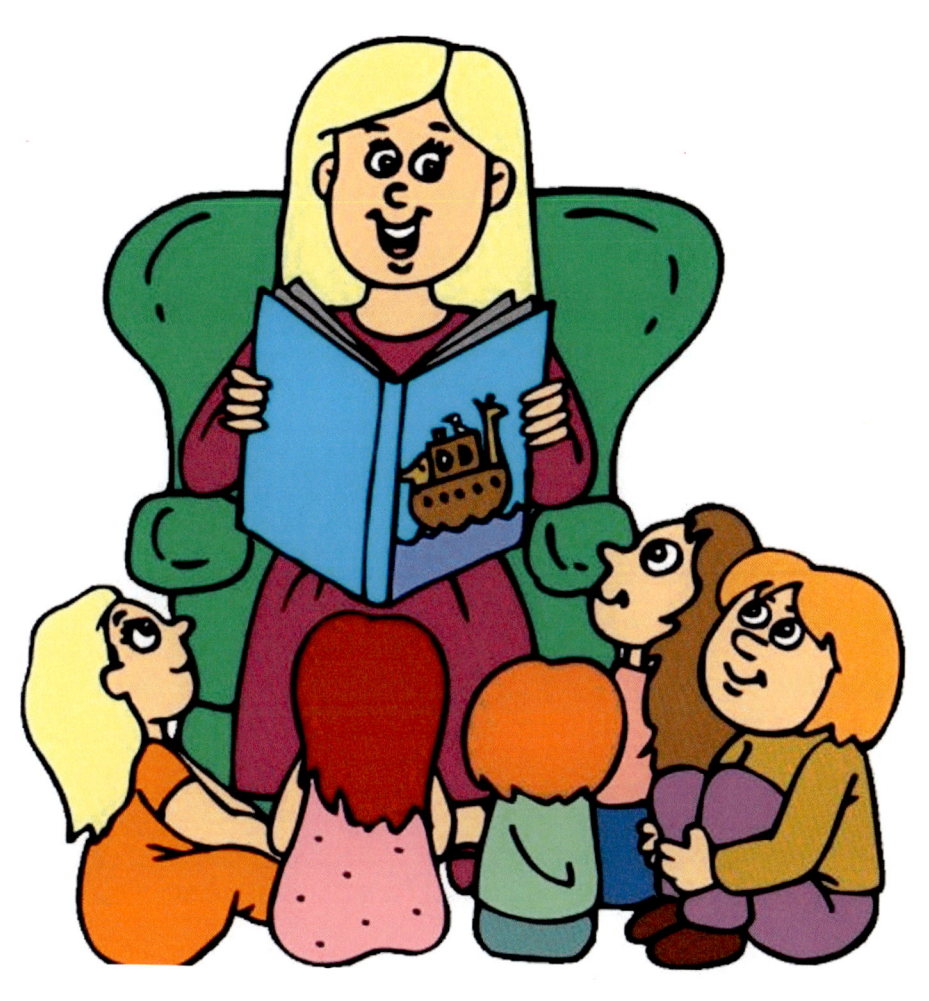

Stories are a great way to describe a scenario in a way that others grasp the concept.

They take various factors into consideration, such as common responses, perspective and social cues in a neatly designed format and style.

There is a huge database of stories available on the internet.

All one needs to do is search for the right term with the right frame of mind.

Frequently Asked Questions

Below are some of the common roadblocks that have been compiled after tireless discussions with parents and professionals who often encounter them while training an autistic child! Further, the questions are arranged with helpful suggestions to help you make the most of this section.

My child has learned to hold if his nappy is not on.

If your child has learned to hold on without his nappies on, it signifies he has a strong bladder. Nevertheless, being consistent will help you achieve the desired results. The child just needs to get accustomed to his new routine.

My child is older than 4 years and shows no signs of toileting

There are rarely signs, if any, for autistic children. One needs to remember that it is all about toilet timing rather than considering the task as toilet training.

No, my child is unable to comply and cannot imitate. What do I do?

Watch out for your child trying to imitate other signs, and if they do, it signals their readiness.

We have met a parent who says they have tried potty training their child and failed. They say they are not interested in retrying to train the child. The child is part of our school.

Consider doing this program yourself. Schedule a consultation with the child's parents. If they are still reluctant about their previous experience, get them to mail us at support@autismag.org

How many bowel movements are ideal for a child every day?
Normally one or two

Nevertheless, have their bowel motions tracked for a week's time before the start of the program.

My child hates the feel of toilet paper
Was your child happy with baby wipes that were used during his nappy days? If so, you can continue using them on the toilet.

My child loves unrolling the toilet paper and makes it a mess every time he visits the toilet.
He loves distractions and loves to play. Remove the toilet paper and give him something else to keep him occupied.

When he has finished, give him toilet paper to clean.

My child acts strangely and loves to completely undress during pooing.
It is normal.

Teach them how to dress and undress on their own.

My child insists on having nappies to do a poo.
Holding bowels can result in constipation. Kiwi crush and kiwi fruit are helpful in such situations.

My child's school bus team insists on nappies being on!
Situations such as these can be tackled with timely discussions. Speak to them and explain your situation. If possible, put a cover on the seat before the child is seated.

When will my child be able to take himself to the toilet?

Success comes in different shapes and forms. Going to the toilet itself is great; many children are unable to do it. Some children never take themselves to the toilet.

At times my child has accidents when he is up to his favorite activity.

Try spending some time to understand his bowel/wee patterns.

Does a ping pong ball help?

It helps to a certain extent. However, when a child has his poo time it can turn out to be a greater mess than otherwise expected. A quick workaround is using bath bombs.

When the child wees in it, it turns out to be a fun movement that children are seen to enjoy.

How do I get my child to wipe his own bottom?

This is something that children will take some time to master. Visuals are a great help to explain things that you might face difficulties with.

Nevertheless, slowly and steadily you can teach your child how to achieve this. This is not a quick task.

Tips for Toileting

1. Understand when your child is ready

Before you even think of starting out the training, use a chart for a week to understand and plot when your child wets his pants. This will help you in understanding the underlying patterns.

2. Using adult toilet

Start with the end goal in mind. Have your child use the toilet right from the beginning. Using alternatives such as potty stairs or potty is an unnecessary burden.

It further helps the child to generalize potty from the toilet and you will see your actions eventually starting to pay off.

3. Toilet timing and not toilet training

Begin with timing your child's toilet activities. Start taking your child every 30 minutes to the toilet and slowly increase the toilet time intervals depending on how they respond to the training sessions.

4. Say no to nappies

Yes! Have a stone heart and say no to nappies. When we say stone heart, remember, you are doing this for the benefit of your child. Small pains lead to success!

5. Night Time Tips

Remember to have the nappy at night, if necessary. Nevertheless, always stick to taking the nappy off as soon as the child gets up in the morning.

You can include a bedtime routine as mentioned below:

- Brushing your child's teeth
- Putting the nappies on
- Wishing goodnight
- Kiss
- Bed

6. Rewards and Positivity

Make the toilet training activity interesting and fun to learn. Combine with rewards that motivate the child to learn more and more.

7. Accidents will happen

It is a normal thing for accidents to happen. Try to be calm and reinforce your training right there. Make the child complete the other tasks such as the toileting routine, flushing, and washing hands.

8. Consider sensory issues

If you find your child having sensory issues, take precautionary measures. Incentivize the child's small achievements.

9. Toilet timing before school age

Try training your child as early as possible. If you neglect early training, you will be faced with increased resistance and hurdles that make toilet training a difficult task.

Keys to Success

- No Nappies
- Consistency
- Routines

Conclusion

It should always be understood that potty training from concept to completion can take years together for a child to master.

Patience and persistence is the key that will pay off eventually.

And when it does, you can pat and congratulate yourself for the job well done!

Nevertheless, success will look different for each and every child, as every child with autism is unique.

Success: Its many Shapes and Forms
- Children will learn to follow adult's prompts. Will wee and poo with lesser accidents.
- The child begins to complete most of the regular routines on their own.
- Children will learn how to successfully use visuals.
- A child gets to know how to follow the steps independently.
- A child learns the art of going to toilet without any prompts in place.

A point worth mentioning: At times, some children are unable to recognize toilet sensations. Some have trouble communicating their need to use the toilet while others have difficulty in having their clothing removed.